CRANIOSACRAL THERAPY

A Comprehensive Guide To Explore The Depths Of Mind-Body Connection, Release Tension, And Restore Balance For Optimal Well-Being

WILFREDO CARSON

INTRODUCTION

Craniosacral Therapy (CST) is a comprehensive approach to healthcare that involves manipulating the craniosacral system, which includes the membranes and cerebrospinal fluid that surround and protect the brain and spinal cord. CST, developed in the early twentieth century by osteopath William Sutherland, is based on the concept that small motions in the craniosacral system can be recognized and managed to improve the body's natural healing processes.

This therapy is based on the concept that the craniosacral rhythm, like the heartbeat and respiration, is a vital physiological function that may be manipulated for therapeutic purposes.

1.1 Background on Craniosacral Therapy:

Craniosacral Therapy has its roots in osteopathy, a type of alternative medicine that focuses on the function of the musculoskeletal system in health and disease. William Sutherland, an American osteopath, made important discoveries in the 1930s that laid the groundwork for CST. He hypothesized that the bones of the skull were not securely bonded, but instead moved in subtle, rhythmic patterns. This resulted in the creation of CST, in which therapists utilize gentle touch to correct abnormalities in the craniosacral system. CST has evolved, incorporating concepts from diverse healing traditions and gaining acceptance as a supplemental therapy for a wide range of ailments.

1.2 Purpose and Scope of the Book:

The goal of this book is to provide a thorough examination of Craniosacral Therapy, including theoretical foundations, practical applications, and evidence supporting its usefulness. It intends to be a beneficial resource for healthcare professionals, students, and anyone who wants to learn about and incorporate CST into their work or personal well-being. The book's scope includes a thorough discussion of the anatomical and physiological concepts that underpin CST, its historical history, and a critical review of its therapeutic uses across a wide range of health issues.

1.3 Targeted Audience:

This book is meant for a wide range of readers, including healthcare practitioners, therapists, students of medicine, osteopathy, and alternative medicine, as well as those seeking a better understanding of Craniosacral Therapy. Professionals seeking to incorporate CST into their practice will find this book to be an invaluable resource, while students will benefit from the in-depth examination of the theoretical and practical components of this therapy. Individuals interested in holistic approaches to health and wellness will also learn about CST's concepts and methodologies.

1.4 How to Use This Book.

To get the most out of this work, readers should use a methodical approach. In the first few chapters, delve into the historical context and theoretical basis of CST. Next, investigate the anatomical and physiological characteristics of the craniosacral system.

The practical implementation of CST techniques is thoroughly discussed, with case examples and research findings to back it up. Readers can go through individual chapters based on their interests, such as learning about the therapeutic benefits of CST for migraines, chronic pain, and stress-related illnesses. The book emphasizes a balanced synthesis of theory and practice to help readers gain a comprehensive understanding of Craniosacral Therapy.

<u>Concepts for Craniosacral Therapy:</u>

CST is based on several basic concepts, each of which is essential for understanding and effectively executing this therapeutic approach. These principles are the

Craniosacral System, Craniosacral Rhythm, Primary Respiratory Mechanism, Inherent Health, and Therapeutic Techniques.

<u>Cranio-sacral System:</u>

Craniosacral Therapy revolves around the craniosacral system, which consists of the membranes and cerebrospinal fluid that surround and protect the brain and spinal cord. This system relies heavily on the dura mater, a thick membrane that surrounds the brain and spinal cord. Therapists use gentle probing to detect and resolve limitations or imbalances in the craniosacral system. Understanding the anatomical components of this system is critical for practitioners seeking to deliver precise and effective therapeutic interventions.

<u>Cranio-sacral rhythm:</u>

The Craniosacral Rhythm, also known as the Primary Respiratory Mechanism, is a faint, repetitive pulse that is thought to be caused by the flow of cerebral spinal fluid. This rhythm is seen as a fundamental representation of life's energy and vitality. CST practitioners use their hands to palpate and evaluate the quality of this rhythm, discovering anomalies or limits. The ability to identify and work with Craniosacral Rhythm is an important talent in CST, as it guides therapists in designing therapies to restore balance and promote healing.

Primary Respiratory Mechanism:

The Primary Respiratory Mechanism refers to the dynamic interaction of the craniosacral system, cranial bones, sacrum, cerebrospinal fluid, and the central nervous system's intrinsic motility. This concept goes beyond physical structures and includes the body's inherent ability to self-regulate and heal. CST acknowledges the intelligence built within this mechanism, stressing the therapist's responsibility to assist and support the body's natural processes rather than imposing external solutions. Understanding the Primary Respiratory Mechanism is essential for therapists to operate in tandem with the body's natural healing abilities.

Inherent Health:

CST is based on the notion of inherent health, which acknowledges the body's fundamental ability to maintain balance and well-being. This concept is consistent with the holistic view that health is more than just the absence of sickness, but a dynamic condition of balance. By eliminating constraints in the craniosacral system, CST strives to improve the body's self-healing capabilities, allowing individuals to achieve inherent health. Craniosacral Therapy is built on a paradigm shift that emphasizes supporting the body's innate resiliency.

<u>Therapeutic techniques:</u>

Craniosacral Therapy involves a variety of therapy modalities to treat specific difficulties with the craniosacral system. These methods involve gentle palpation, discreet manipulations, and positional holds. Practitioners use their hands to discover and release limitations, which aids in the restoration of balance and optimal function. These approaches need precision, sensitivity, and a thorough understanding of anatomy and physiology.

Throughout the book, extensive explanations and illustrations help readers grasp these therapeutic approaches, emphasizing the need to take a gentle and non-invasive approach.

<u>Clinical applications:</u>

Craniosacral Therapy has clinical implications for a variety of health issues, including both physical and mental well-being. Extensive research and case studies demonstrate the effectiveness of CST in treating migraines, chronic pain, stress-related problems, and neurodevelopmental abnormalities. The book dives deeply into each application, examining the underlying mechanics and evidence-based outcomes. Furthermore, it investigates the integration of CST with traditional medical methods, highlighting the potential for collaborative and complementary approaches to improve overall patient care.

This book offers a thorough overview of Craniosacral Therapy, with in-depth discussions of its theory, procedures, and clinical applications. CST is a one-of-a-kind approach to healthcare that highlights the body's natural healing abilities. It is based on a comprehensive study of the craniosacral system and its rhythmic expressions.

The book is designed to appeal to a wide range of readers, including healthcare professionals, students, and others interested in holistic well-being. This book intends to contribute to the continuous discourse and progress of CST within the larger healthcare landscape by instilling a deep respect for its principles and practices.

CHAPTER 1
FOUNDATIONS OF CRANIOSACRAL THERAPY

Definition and history of Craniosacral Therapy:

Craniosacral Therapy (CST) is a comprehensive approach to healthcare that focuses on the intricate movements of the cranial bones, sacrum, and cerebrospinal fluid inside the central nervous system. CST, which originated in osteopathy, was established by Dr. John E. Upledger in the 1970s when he discovered previously unknown rhythmic movements of the cranial sutures. The therapy uses gentle touch and manipulation of the craniosacral system to boost the body's natural healing capacities. Dr. William Sutherland, an osteopathic physician, pioneered the concept of cranial bone movement in the early twentieth century. CST has subsequently evolved into a unique therapy with its own set of ideas and practices, earning acceptance in both complementary and conventional healthcare settings.

<u>Principles and philosophy:</u>

Craniosacral Therapy's main ideas are based on the belief that the body has an innate potential to repair itself. The therapy is based on the idea that the craniosacral system, which includes the membranes and cerebrospinal fluid that surround and protect the brain and spinal cord, moves in a rhythmic pattern. This tiny motion, known as craniosacral rhythm, is thought to be essential for overall health and well-being. CST practitioners follow this rhythm, utilizing light touch and expert probing to assess and correct any limitations or imbalances in the craniosacral system.

The therapy emphasizes the interconnectedness of the body, mind, and spirit, and sees the individual as a dynamic entity. The concept also believes that facilitating the craniosacral rhythm might improve the body's self-regulation systems.

<u>Historical Development:</u>

Craniosacral Therapy has a rich history, dating back to Dr. William Sutherland's early concepts of cranial mobility. His observations of the repetitive motion of the cranial bones paved the way for what would become CST. However, Dr. John E. Upledger established and perfected the therapy in the 1970s. Upledger, an osteopathic physician, elaborated on Sutherland's concepts and established the concept of craniosacral rhythm as a therapeutic approach. His work resulted in the formation of the Upledger Institute, a well-known institution that educates and develops CST practitioners around the world. Craniosacral Therapy has grown in popularity over the years, transitioning from its osteopathic roots to an independent therapy used by a wide range of healthcare practitioners.

Anatomy and Physiology Related to the Craniosacral System:

Craniosacral Therapy requires a thorough understanding of the craniosacral system's anatomy and physiology. The system includes the membranes (meninges) that surround the brain and spinal cord, as well as the cerebrospinal fluid that circulates within the enclosed space. The key components are the dura mater, arachnoid mater, and pia mater, which house and protect the central nervous system. The cerebrospinal fluid produced in the brain's ventricles circulates through the subarachnoid space, resulting in a modest rhythmic motion known as craniosacral rhythm. CST practitioners feel that the rhythm indicates the nerve system's vigor and wellness. The therapy consists of hands-on procedures designed to alleviate limits or tensions in the craniosacral system, allowing for optimal movement of cerebrospinal fluid and increasing overall well-being. Craniosacral Therapy's precise and gentle manipulations are based on a thorough grasp of the complex anatomy and physiology of the craniosacral system.

CHAPTER 2
THE CRANIOSACRAL SYSTEM

The craniosacral system is an essential part of the human anatomy and physiology, helping to preserve health and balance. This system includes the cranium, or skull, and the sacrum, a triangle bone at the base of the spine. These components are linked by the dura mater, a protective membrane that surrounds the brain and spinal cord. They constitute a continuous system that is essential to the functioning of the central nervous system. The craniosacral system is central to craniosacral therapy, a holistic therapeutic approach that addresses the system's delicate movements and rhythms.

<u>Understanding Cranial Sacral Rhythm:</u>

The craniosacral rhythm is a faint, regular pulsing that can be palpated throughout the body. This rhythm is due to the generation and reabsorption of cerebrospinal fluid, which surrounds and protects the brain and spinal cord. The craniosacral rhythm is said to reflect an individual's innate health and vitality, with disturbances indicating imbalances or constraints in the craniosacral system. Craniosacral therapy practitioners use their hands to detect and evaluate this rhythm, which allows them to pinpoint regions of stress or dysfunction while also facilitating the body's self-healing mechanisms.

<u>The Craniosacral System includes the following components:</u>

The craniosacral system is made up of numerous critical components that work together to promote an individual's overall well-being. The skull, made up of cranial bones and sutures, serves as the brain's protective encasement. The spine, which runs from the base of the skull to the sacrum, houses the spinal cord. The dura mater is a strong membrane that surrounds the brain and spinal cord, connecting the cranium and sacrum. Additionally, cerebrospinal fluid circulates throughout the dura mater, feeding and cushioning the central nervous system. Understanding the interplay of these components is critical in craniosacral treatment, as practitioners aim to improve the body's ability to self-regulate and heal.

<u>Cerebrospinal Fluid and Its Function:</u>

Cerebrospinal fluid (CSF) is a clear, colorless fluid found in the brain's ventricles, the subarachnoid space, and the spinal cord's central canal. It performs a variety of important roles within the craniosacral system. One of its key functions is to serve as a protective cushion, absorbing shocks and preventing injury to fragile neural tissues. Furthermore, CSF supports the flow of nutrients and waste products between the blood and neural tissue, helping to support the central nervous system's general metabolic function. Craniosacral treatment meticulously assesses and addresses the flow and balance of cerebrospinal fluid to promote optimal functioning and alleviate any constraints that may obstruct its circulation.

<u>Cranial bones and sutures:</u>

The cranial bones and sutures are essential components of the craniosacral system, which forms the bony framework that surrounds and protects the brain. The human skull is made up of several bones: the frontal, parietal, temporal, occipital, sphenoid, and ethmoid. Sutures connect these bones, and fibrous joints allow for some flexibility and mobility.

The movement at these sutures is not only necessary for the birthing process but it is also considered an important component of the craniosacral rhythm. Craniosacral therapy practitioners focus on the subtle motions and tensions within the cranial bones and sutures, to release constraints and restore normal mobility. The complicated interplay between these bones and sutures is crucial for the normal operation of the craniosacral system and, by extension, the individual's overall health.

To summarize, the craniosacral system is a complex and integrated network in the human body that includes the cranium, sacrum, cerebrospinal fluid, and cranial bones with sutures. Understanding craniosacral rhythm and the role of cerebrospinal fluid serves as the foundation for craniosacral treatment, a holistic approach that aims to improve the body's self-healing capabilities. By treating imbalances and constraints in the craniosacral system, practitioners hope to promote optimal health and well-being. The craniosacral system's complicated dynamics highlight its importance in the larger context of human anatomy, as well as the possibility of therapeutic intervention to support and improve its function.

CHAPTER 3
CRANIOSACRAL THERAPY TECHNIQUES

Craniosacral Therapy (CST) is a gentle and holistic treatment technique that focuses on manipulating the craniosacral system, which includes the membranes and cerebrospinal fluid that surround and protect the brain and spinal cord. This therapy includes a variety of approaches, each with a distinct goal of enhancing overall well-being and treating various physical and emotional disorders.

In this exploration, we gain a thorough understanding of the fundamental concepts and practices that comprise Craniosacral Therapy.

Evaluation and Assessment Methods

Observation and palpation are critical components of the evaluation procedure in Craniosacral Therapy. Practitioners carefully examine the client's posture, motions, and overall demeanor to get insight into the body's state. Palpation, or the skill of feeling with the hands, enables therapists to discover subtle rhythms, limitations, and imbalances in the craniosacral system. This hands-on technique enables practitioners to detect areas of stress or dysfunction, establishing the framework for focused therapeutic approaches.

Listening and sensing are essential abilities in the practitioner's repertoire, allowing the therapist to recognize the body's natural rhythms and variations. Craniosacral Therapy practitioners become aware of the craniosacral rhythm, which is a gentle pulsation caused by the movement of CSF fluids.

Using acute hearing and feeling skills, therapists can discover anomalies in this rhythm and customize interventions to restore balance and reduce constraints.

Craniosacral Therapy requires a thorough awareness of anatomical landmarks to provide proper assessment and intervention. Practitioners explore the complex topography of the craniosacral system, identifying essential components and their interactions.

This knowledge forms the basis for precise palpation and manipulation, ensuring that treatment efforts are focused and effective. Mastery of anatomical markers enables practitioners to navigate the complex craniosacral system with precision and confidence.

Basic Craniosacral Techniques

The Still Point Technique is a trademark of Craniosacral Therapy, designed to produce deep relaxation and release within the craniosacral system. This technique includes gently cradling the head or sacrum to temporarily interrupt the craniosacral rhythm. This pause, or "still point," allows stored tension to evaporate, resulting in a deep sense of relaxation. The Still Point Technique is strategically used to treat diseases connected with craniosacral abnormalities, providing a therapeutic environment for the body to self-correct and heal.

Soft Tissue Release in Craniosacral Therapy is the gentle and deliberate manipulation of soft tissues to relieve tension and limitations. Practitioners utilize delicate motions to relieve tension or adhesions in the connective tissues that surround the craniosacral system.

This approach promotes increased mobility, lowers pain, and improves general function in the affected areas. Soft Tissue Release is very effective for treating musculoskeletal disorders and establishing a more fluid craniosacral rhythm.

Energy Balancing is a comprehensive approach to Craniosacral Therapy that recognizes the interdependence of the physical and energetic parts of the body. Practitioners use their intention and awareness to encourage the free flow of energy through the craniosacral system. This approach uses gentle touch and energetic awareness to detect and treat blockages or interruptions in the body's energy flow. Energy Balancing seeks to restore harmony on both the physical and energy levels, promoting a sense of balance and vitality.

Advanced Techniques and Modalities

Somatoemotional release (SER) is a more sophisticated Craniosacral Therapy practice that addresses the interconnectedness of physical and emotional sensations.

This technique acknowledges that trauma and emotional stress can show as physical limits in the craniosacral system. SER entails leading the client through a process of exploring and releasing buried emotional patterns housed in the tissues. By encouraging the integration of emotional and physical experiences, SER supports deep healing and the resolution of both physical and emotional issues.

Visceral Manipulation is a Craniosacral Therapy technique that involves manipulating the internal organs to improve their movement and function. Practitioners use gentle, targeted touch to treat limitations or imbalances in the visceral tissues. This technique identifies the numerous linkages between organs and surrounding systems, with the goal of optimizing organ function and promoting general health. Visceral manipulation is particularly beneficial for treating organ dysfunction, digestive difficulties, and pelvic health.

Pediatrics Craniosacral Therapy applies the principles of Craniosacral Therapy to the specific needs of newborns and children.

This specialist approach recognizes how birth trauma, developmental problems, and other variables affect a child's well-being. Practitioners use gentle, non-invasive approaches to promote the healthy development of the craniosacral system in paediatric patients. Pediatrics Craniosacral Therapy is effective in treating issues such as colic, breastfeeding difficulties, and developmental delays, laying the groundwork for optimal health from a young age.

Craniosacral Therapy includes a diverse set of procedures based on careful evaluation, nuanced palpation, and an awareness of the body's complex anatomical environment. From core diagnostic methods to advanced modalities, Craniosacral Therapy promotes holistic well-being and addresses a wide range of physical and emotional disorders.

The blending of these approaches exemplifies Craniosacral Therapy's therapeutic creativity, building a deep connection between practitioner and client on the path to optimal health.

CHAPTER 4
CONDITIONS AND INDICATIONS FOR CRANIOSACRAL THERAPY

Craniosacral therapy (CST) is a comprehensive approach to healthcare that focuses on manipulating and balancing the craniosacral system, which includes the membranes and cerebrospinal fluid that surround the brain and spinal cord. This therapy technique is well-known for its adaptability and effectiveness in treating a wide range of health issues. The next paragraphs go into detail about CST's therapeutic applications in a variety of fields.

Pain Management: One of Craniosacral Therapy's core uses is pain management. CST practitioners emphasize the importance of the craniosacral system in sustaining overall health, and interruptions in its rhythm are thought to lead to pain and discomfort.

The mild manipulations used during CST sessions are intended to alleviate tension in the connective tissues around the central nervous system, promoting relaxation and pain relief. Migraines, tension headaches, and chronic pain syndromes have been found to improve with regular CST sessions. CST's subtle but significant effects on the nervous system make it an appealing alternative for people seeking non-invasive pain alleviation.

Stress and Anxiety: Craniosacral Therapy is also used as a therapeutic therapy to treat stress and anxiety. The craniosacral system regulates the autonomic nerve system, which controls the body's stress reaction. CST uses gentle touch and manipulation to regulate the craniosacral rhythm, allowing for deep relaxation. This relaxation response can help to counterbalance the chronic activation of the stress response found in those suffering from anxiety disorders. Clients frequently express feelings of relaxation and enhanced mental well-being after CST sessions. This therapy's comprehensive approach, which addresses both physical and emotional components, makes it an effective complement to traditional stress management treatments.

Neurological illnesses: Craniosacral Therapy has been investigated as a complementary method to the treatment of several neurological illnesses. While not a replacement for medical therapies, CST is thought to affect the central nervous system, potentially aiding in symptom control. CST practitioners have expressed an interest in conditions such as multiple sclerosis, Parkinson's disease, and cerebral palsy. The gentle manipulations are thought to increase cerebrospinal fluid flow, which may impact neuronal function. It is important to emphasize that research in this field is continuing, and the incorporation of CST into neurological care regimens should be carried out under the supervision of healthcare professionals.

Trauma rehabilitation: Craniosacral Therapy is well-known for its involvement in physical and mental trauma rehabilitation. Muscular tension, restricted movement, and emotional anguish are some of the physical manifestations of trauma. CST practitioners approach trauma from a comprehensive standpoint, recognizing the interdependence of physical and emotional well-being.

The gentle touch utilized in CST sessions tries to remove constraints in the fascia and nervous system, which may aid in the treatment of trauma symptoms. Individuals who have sustained physical injuries, accidents, or mental trauma may find CST to be an important part of their overall recovery strategy.

Pediatrics disorders: Craniosacral Therapy is deemed safe for children and is commonly used to treat a variety of paediatric disorders. Parents seek CST for a variety of reasons, including birth trauma, developmental difficulties, and conditions like colic and sleep disturbances. Practitioners utilize a gentle touch to diagnose and treat any constraints in the craniosacral system that may be affecting a child's health. Pediatrics CST research is expanding, with some trials showing promising results in disorders such as infantile colic. Parents must speak with healthcare specialists and certified CST practitioners to ensure that the therapy is appropriate for their child's unique requirements.

Other Health Issues: Aside from the specific categories stated, Craniosacral Therapy is used to treat a wide range of health problems. CST is being studied as a supplementary therapy for gastrointestinal diseases, immune system dysfunction, and respiratory illnesses. CST's holistic approach, which takes into account the interconnectivity of multiple biological systems, is thought to contribute to its versatility in dealing with a wide range of health conditions. While research in some of these areas is still ongoing, anecdotal evidence and clinical observations frequently emphasize the potential benefits of CST in terms of overall health and well-being.

Craniosacral Therapy provides a comprehensive and non-invasive approach to healthcare, with applications spanning from pain treatment to pediatric care. The subtle but substantial effects on the craniosacral system are thought to affect a variety of physiological and psychological processes. As with any therapy modality, patients must consult with experienced healthcare providers to evaluate whether Craniosacral Therapy is appropriate for their requirements. Ongoing research and investigation into its mechanisms help to better grasp the potential benefits and limitations of this therapy strategy across a wide range of health issues.

CHAPTER 5
INTEGRATING CRANIOSACRAL THERAPY INTO HEALTH CARE

Craniosacral therapy (CST) has gained popularity as a holistic approach to healthcare, emphasizing the interconnectivity of the body's systems and the possibility of self-healing. Integrating CST into mainstream healthcare necessitates working with other healthcare providers to provide full patient care. The combination of CST and traditional treatment can be especially effective in tackling complex health concerns. Healthcare practitioners can enhance multidisciplinary communication and understanding, resulting in a more inclusive and patient-centered approach that recognizes the significance of both standard medical interventions and complementary therapies.

Collaboration with Other Healthcare Professionals.

Effective collaboration with other healthcare experts is critical to the effective integration of Craniosacral Therapy into traditional healthcare settings. This relationship requires open communication, mutual respect, and a shared commitment to patient well-being. Interdisciplinary discussions, joint training sessions, and collaborative research initiatives can help CST practitioners and mainstream healthcare providers communicate more effectively. This collaboration will provide healthcare practitioners with insights into the concepts and advantages of CST, allowing them to make more educated decisions about its inclusion in treatment programs. Such collaborations can also contribute to a more comprehensive understanding of patients' needs, resulting in better health outcomes.

Research and Evidence-Based Practices

The incorporation of Craniosacral Therapy into healthcare necessitates a strong dedication to research and evidence-based treatment. While CST has a history based on holistic concepts, proving its efficacy through scientific research is critical to getting widespread recognition in the medical field. Robust clinical studies, systematic reviews, and meta-analyses can provide empirical evidence for CST's therapeutic benefits. This study not only strengthens the legitimacy of CST, but also educates healthcare practitioners on its unique applications, contraindications, and potential hazards. Evidence-based practice guarantees that CST is implemented in healthcare in a responsible and informed manner, by modern medical care standards.

Ethical considerations

As Craniosacral Therapy becomes more widely used in healthcare, ethical considerations are critical to ensure patient safety and well-being. Practitioners must follow a rigorous code of ethics that controls their dealings with patients, coworkers, and the larger healthcare community. Transparency in treatment methods, informed permission, and safeguarding patient anonymity are all critical ethical considerations in CST. Furthermore, practitioners must be aware of their scope of practice and interact with other healthcare experts as needed. Ethical principles help to establish CST's credibility in the healthcare system and promote a patient-centered approach that values the individual's autonomy and right to make informed decisions about their healthcare journey.

Case Studies & Success Stories

Documenting and sharing case studies and success stories is an essential component of incorporating Craniosacral Therapy into healthcare. These narratives serve several functions: they provide real-world examples of CST applications, insights into treatment outcomes, and help to construct a corpus of experience knowledge. Case examples demonstrate CST's adaptability in addressing a wide range of health concerns, including chronic pain and emotional well-being. Success stories not only boost patient confidence but also provide healthcare personnel with actual instances of CST's positive influence. By spreading such anecdotal evidence, the healthcare community can gain a better understanding of CST's potential advantages and help it integrate into mainstream care.

Integrating Craniosacral Therapy into healthcare requires a complex strategy that includes collaboration with other healthcare professionals, a dedication to research and evidence-based treatment, ethical considerations, and the documentation of case studies and success stories. As the lines between conventional and complementary medicine become increasingly blurred, integrating holistic therapies such as CST can help to create a more comprehensive and patient-centered healthcare system. Integrating CST into mainstream healthcare through open discourse, rigorous research, and a commitment to ethical behavior has the potential to improve overall patient well-being and broaden the frontiers of current medical care.

CHAPTER 6
TRAINING AND CERTIFICATION IN CRANIOSACRAL THERAPY

Craniosacral Therapy (CST) is a specific type of bodywork that focuses on the craniosacral system, which includes the membranes and cerebrospinal fluid that surround the brain and spinal cord. Educational programs and schools that provide Craniosacral Therapy training play an important role in developing competent practitioners in this profession. These schools often offer a thorough curriculum that includes anatomy, physiology, and hands-on practical skills. Students explore the complexities of the craniosacral system, learning to recognize subtle motions and rhythms that affect general health. Institutions that offer such programs differ in their approaches, with some emphasizing a more biomechanical perspective and others incorporating a holistic outlook.

The individual practitioner's interests and aims within the field of Craniosacral Therapy frequently influence the program selection.

Certification Requirements: Becoming certified in Craniosacral Therapy is an important step for practitioners looking to build reputation and proficiency in the profession. Certification requirements act as benchmarks to verify that therapists satisfy specific levels of knowledge and skill. These guidelines are often established by respectable certifying bodies or groups committed to upholding the integrity of Craniosacral Therapy practice. Certification programs often include a mix of theoretical evaluations, practical exams, and recorded clinical experience.

Educational qualifications from authorized institutions are frequently required, ensuring that licensed practitioners have a strong understanding of anatomy, physiology, and Craniosacral Therapy concepts. Some certification boards may also require candidates to complete a certain number of supervised clinical hours to demonstrate their competency in implementing the therapy in a real-world setting.

Continuing Education & Professional Development: In the ever-changing area of healthcare, Craniosacral Therapy practitioners must stay current on developing trends, refine their abilities, and maintain a high level of care. Continuing education programs allow therapists to expand their knowledge of advanced procedures, investigate particular areas of Craniosacral Therapy, and participate in interdisciplinary studies. These studies may include advanced anatomy, neurobiology, and the incorporation of Craniosacral Therapy with other modalities. Furthermore, professional development may include workshops, conferences, and seminars that allow therapists to exchange ideas, debate difficult situations, and expand their network within the healthcare community. Continuous learning not only improves the expertise of Craniosacral Therapy practitioners, but it also helps to advance and establish the field's legitimacy in the larger healthcare environment.

the Craniosacral Therapy education and certification environment is complex and ever-changing.

Educational programs and schools lay the groundwork for a practitioner's knowledge; certification standards establish the norm for competency; and continuous education assures continual growth and relevance in the area. As practitioners navigate this complex landscape, they help to further the growth and acknowledgment of Craniosacral Therapy as a valued and acknowledged therapy in the field of complementary and alternative medicine.

CHAPTER SEVEN

BEYOND THE BASICS: PERSONAL EXPERIENCES AND INSIGHTS

1. Interviews with Experienced Craniosacral Therapists:

When diving beyond the fundamentals of Craniosacral Therapy (CST), it is critical to consider the perspectives of experienced practitioners in the area. Interviews with these experienced therapists give insight into the finer points of CST that go beyond textbook knowledge. These specialists, typically with years of hands-on experience, offer a unique perspective on the complexities of treatment. Through their stories, one can learn not only the technical parts of the field but also the subtle nuances that come with years of experience working with a variety of people and conditions.

Experienced Craniosacral Therapists frequently explain the growth of their technique throughout time. These interviews reveal how practitioners modify and improve their strategies, incorporating new knowledge and insights into their sessions. The interviews also shed light on the problems that therapists confront, such as dealing with complex cases and handling the emotional aspects of their employment. Furthermore, investigating the therapists' perspectives on the larger field of complementary and alternative medicine improves our awareness of the interdependence of diverse holistic healing approaches.

<u>Two client testimonials:</u>

Client testimonies demonstrate the effectiveness of Craniosacral Therapy for those seeking its benefits. These accounts add a qualitative dimension to the efficacy of CST, providing insight into the lived experiences of persons who have received the therapy. Clients describe in detail how CST transformed their physical, emotional, and mental well-being.

Testimonials frequently focus on specific ailments or disorders for which customers sought help, as well as how Craniosacral Therapy aided in their recovery. The range of illnesses treated - from chronic pain to stress-related problems - demonstrates CST's adaptability as a therapeutic method. Exploring these testimonials also sheds light on the subjective nature of healing, as clients express not just physical changes but also shifts in their general quality of life and sense of self.

Client testimonies also contribute to the ongoing discussion about the safety and ethical implications of Craniosacral Therapy. knowledge of the experiences of persons who have used CST helps to assess the possible benefits and limitations of the therapy in various circumstances, resulting in a more complete knowledge of its consequences.

3. Personal Reflections on the Practice:

Personal insights from practitioners provide valuable insight into the inner workings of Craniosacral Therapy. Therapists frequently participate in introspective evaluation, reflecting on their progress, problems, and the symbiotic relationship that develops between therapist and client.

These comments provide insight into the practice's emotional and spiritual elements, in addition to the palpable physical skills.

Exploring personal perspectives reveals therapists' deep connection to the delicate rhythms and energies encountered during CST sessions. These insights dive into the intuitive parts of the therapy, in which therapists discuss connecting with the body's natural wisdom and aiding a self-directed healing process. Such views add to the ongoing discussion about the holistic nature of Craniosacral Therapy, which goes beyond the mechanical components to include the connectivity of mind, body, and spirit.

Furthermore, personal reflections frequently address the ethical implications and duties that come with practicing CST.

Therapists discuss building trust with clients, preserving professional boundaries, and striking the difficult balance between intuition and evidence-based practice. These insights are an excellent resource for both new and seasoned practitioners, encouraging a culture of ongoing learning and ethical self-examination within the Craniosacral Therapy community.

CONCLUSION

Craniosacral Therapy develops as a diverse and dynamic healing method that goes beyond the limitations of traditional medical approaches. Beyond the fundamental ideas and practices, insights gathered from interviews with experienced therapists, client testimonials, and personal reflections on the practice all add to a more complete understanding of CST.

The interviews with seasoned practitioners highlight the evolution and adaptation of the field, demonstrating how experience refines therapeutic approaches.

Client testimonials, on the other hand, tell powerful stories of healing, emphasizing CST's ability to treat a wide range of diseases and the subjective aspect of well-being. Therapists' perspectives illuminate the intuitive and spiritual components of their work, emphasizing the interdependence of mind, body, and spirit in the healing process.

This thorough investigation emphasizes the importance of CST in the field of complementary and alternative medicine.

It highlights the importance of ongoing research, ethical considerations, and a comprehensive approach to health and wellness. Craniosacral Therapy, with its subtle yet powerful effects, continues to attract both practitioners and clients, creating a rich tapestry of experiences that add to the ever-changing landscape of holistic therapy.